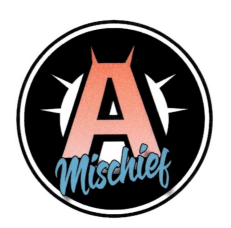

The Absolute Beginner's Guide to...Domination

By Mistress Max Absolute

Illustrations by Satine Phoenix

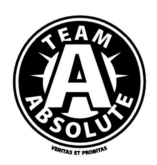

First published in Great Britain 2015

Second Edition in 2020
By Absolute Mischief Ltd
www.absolutebeginnersguide.co.uk

Copyright © 2015, 2020 by Max Absolute

All rights reserved. No part of this book may be reproduced or utilised in any form or means, electronic or mechanical, including photocopying, recording or by any information storage and retrieval system, without written permission.

A catalogue record for this book is available from the British Library

Design by Rachel May
Illustrations by Satine Phoenix
About the Author photo by Rebecca Seal-Davies
Back cover photo by Kate Peters

ISBN-13: 978-1507880265
ISBN-10: 150788026X

This book is dedicated to all the amazing Dominant Ladies who over the years have taught Me so much and who have been so much fun to be around.

You know who You are.....

Contents

Introduction 9

Chapter 1
Where Do I Start? 12
Why Domination? 13
Things to remember 14
Key points 15
Rules of Conduct 17
Taking Control 22
What is a Dom(me)? 23
The Sub/Dom relationship 25
Care involved in being Dominant 26

Chapter 2
Finding Your Style of Domination 29
Dominant Characters 30
What's Dominant about them? 31
Your Dominant style 32
Methods of Domination 33

Chapter 3
Introducing Domination into your relationship 35
Bringing up the subject 37
Who plays which role? 39
Creating the ground rules 40

Chapter 4
Equipment 41
Using yourself! 42
Basic toys 43
Outfits and fetish fashion 46

Chapter 5
Games, Scenes & Planning 47
Now what? 48
Planning ahead 50
Games to get you started 55

Chapter 6
Out & About 62
Clubs and Events 63
Finding a playmate 65

Further Reading 67

Annual Events 68

Glossary 70

About the Author 77

"Man is the one who desires, woman the one who is desired. This is woman's entire but decisive advantage. Through his passion nature has given man into woman's hands, and the woman who does not know how to make him her subject, her slave, her toy, and how to betray him with a smile in the end is not wise."

Leopold von Sacher-Masoch, *Venus in Furs*

Introduction

Having been a professional and lifestyle Dominatrix for over a decade, I delight in sharing the art of Domination as well as practising it. Domination is about taking the lead in your playtime. This book is designed to give you the skills to take that lead........

One of the most common misunderstandings is that domination is just about hurting another person; in fact there are many ways to express dominance other than simply causing someone pain. From a discreet whispered order in public, or selecting your partner's outfit for a date night, right through to a stinging thwack from the crop. What they have in common is that taking control of a lover, with their consent of course, offers a deliciously decadent pleasure. While I've contributed to numerous books on fetish over the years, I've often been disappointed by fetish and sex authors' tendencies to over-complicate the subject — which is where the Absolute Beginner's Guides come in.

With society becoming much more accepting and open about sex, it has in turn highlighted the huge variety of things that people can, and do, find sexually stimulating. The Internet has provided an anonymous space to demonstrate the extent to which indulging in this huge variety of kinky pleasures actually happens. You are not alone or odd in wanting to give this a go.

The Internet has revealed just how diverse the world of sexual tastes actually is. To some the Internet allows them to find likeminded people, and for others it opens up new possibilities and options to explore their own sexuality. The flip side is that so much choice can be daunting and overwhelming and with some imagery pushing the boundaries of what is real and safe to a point where the lines of reality and fantasy are so blurred and extreme that they're inaccessible for most.

People post all sorts of pictures and clips online, and although there are many sites online that are fetish videos and pictures made by women, the majority of them are still made for men featuring model-like female Dommes engaging in very harsh extreme play with the submissive in apparent great pain or looking desperately unhappy. This offers an unrealistic representation and can be so off-putting to anyone looking for a lighter or more fun style of Domination and sometimes they can be slightly intimidating to anyone outside of the fetish model standard of looks and body shape.

Whatever path led to you picking up this book, take comfort in the fact that you are not alone, and remember that we all started out as novices and the process of learning and developing never ends unless you want it to! Some of the things you may decide to try won't be something that works for you, some you may find are things you like to indulge in every now and then, or you may find are a whole new way of expressing your sexual and sometimes non-sexual personality. Everyone is different and therefore your style and preferences should reflect that. The only person who can decide that for you is YOU...

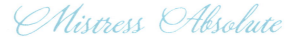

Mistress Absolute

Chapter One

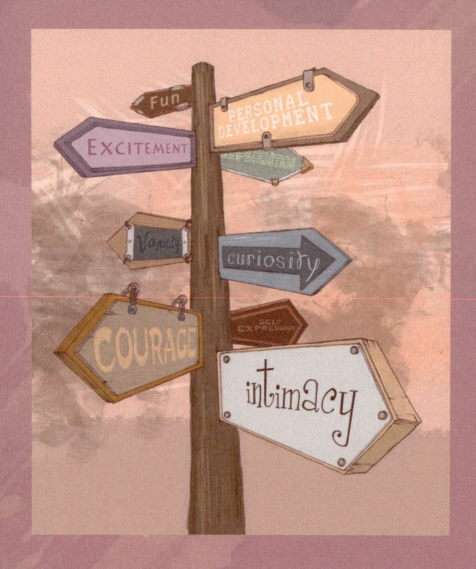

Where do I start?

Why Domination?

Exploring a Dominant play style can add to your existing sex life, spice it up or add some variety. But it can also help you find alternative facets of your personality.

People often panic when trying to find a starting point to explore and discover what domination & submission might mean or offer them, but once you understand a few core concepts you can creatively explore your personal Dominant desires.

Most people have exactly the same questions and concerns when they start. The pressure of getting it "right" can sometimes be so overpowering it's easy to forget some obvious but vital things about what you are doing.

Here are some things to keep in mind when starting out that should help you from panicking!

Things to Remember

1. It should be fun!
2. This is YOUR own personal adventure of self-discovery.
3. This is something you should be doing for yourself or trying it because you want to give it a go.
4. This should not be an unpleasant pressure to become someone else's fantasy.
5. It's perfectly fine to like some things you try and it's totally all right <u>not</u> to like some things you try.
6. Not everything is going to feel immediately "natural."
7. It's OK to find things funny.
8. Communication and honesty are vital.
9. Don't be pressured into doing something you don't want to do or are not ready to try yet.
10. And I am going to repeat this one, because it's the most frequently forgotten but most vital point…

IT'S SUPPOSED TO BE FUN!!

Key points

Let me reveal a key point to further remove any last bits of self-inflicted pressure: as long as you are not ending up in a place that is mentally or physically unsafe for you or the person(s) you are with then there are no right or wrongs. It's all about finding a style and approach you feel comfortable with; and don't be afraid to develop, change or try new or variations of your Domme self.

Everyone makes mistakes, has an off-day, or experiences things that just don't go as well as you thought they would in your head, and it's OK to admit that! Don't be afraid to communicate with your partner and discuss what you might both change for the better next time.

As you might have picked up on, most people call this "play" for a very good reason; play is associated with a fun unpressured time where the seriousness of everyday pressures are suspended and where you get to make up the rules. Sometimes it's good to remind yourself that playing is fun and the rules of the game are yours to set, and your imagination is the only limit!

There's no single Dominant personality — even the most submissive person may be surprised to find an inner Dom(me) lurking deep inside. You don't need to be scared of "doing it wrong," fetish play should be fun, not a chore. And there is no ABC of Domination — but by gaining an Absolute foundation to Domination, you can develop your own unique style.

This book is for anyone who would like to explore taking control. It does not matter if you don't consider yourself a naturally dominant person in or out of the bedroom; this guide is designed to let you play in a leading role and feel comfortable doing it.

So if you are ready to play, have fun and find your inner-Dominant then read on!

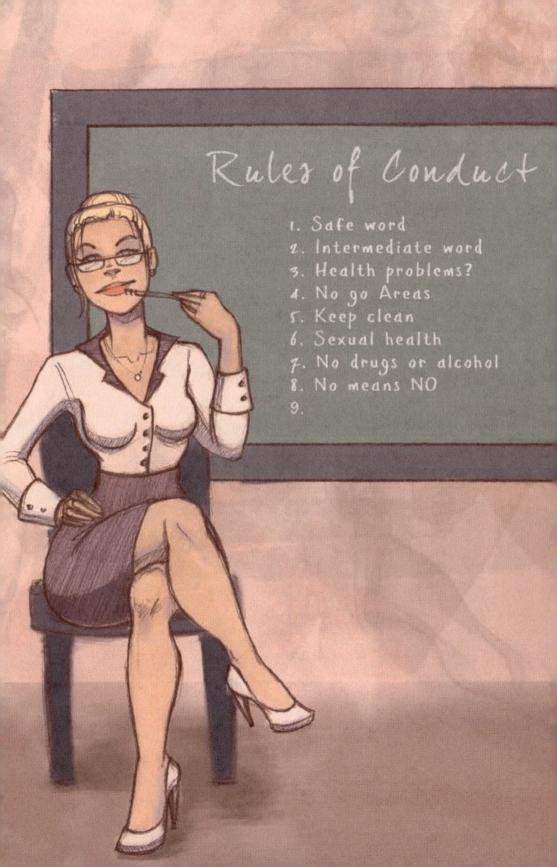

Rules of Conduct

It is good to make sure that whatever sort of play you engage in you do so in a safe, sane and consensual manner. It may seem boring or passion-killing, but it's the essential foundation and by covering everything beforehand, it makes for safe, fun play with no misunderstandings. Below is a short check-list of things which should be addressed prior to play:

- The safe word. Pick a word that you would not usually use in the bedroom or playroom such as red or banana and communicate to each other that that is the safe word for play. If either of you say the safe word the play stops immediately. It should only be used if there is an emergency.
- Intermediate safe word. It may be useful, especially when you start playing with someone, to have an intermediate safe word, a "time out" word so to speak. This gives you both room to communicate open and honestly while you learn about each other. If you use red as your safe-word you may like to use amber as your intermediate safe-word — "time out" works well too!

The safe words are there to protect both of you to be sure that you can communicate quickly and clearly if there is a serious problem. Once the safe word is in place, you both are free to safely lose yourself in your fantasy.

- Health problems. Not every health issue is easy to see (asthma, heart conditions, etc.) so it is imperative that you check with your partner if there are any health problems that they might have before you start playing. It is also good to know about any medications your partner might be taking as you may need to take into account how these may impede your partner's ability to make balanced decisions. Additionally ask about allergies; the last thing you want is to put on a new latex dress only to find out your play partner is allergic to it!

- Sexual health. You don't have to have full intercourse to pick up something nasty — oral contact can land you with many an STI. Have regular sexual health checks yourself and discuss your partner's sexual health with them to keep them and yourself safe. Use protection. Have ample supplies. Educate yourself about what is out there and how you can protect yourself by popping into your local clinic or checking an online, reputable site or two.

- Be aware of the risks. If you don't know how to do something it's probably better you don't just "have a go." Find out as much as you can about what you want to do and the risks involved before you try.

- » No go areas. You may have a very clear idea of the things you may or may not want to get up to when playing but it may not be the same list of things for your partner. Communication is key, so make sure you discuss your boundaries in advance. Boundaries may shift over time so take care to discuss and update your lists from time to time.

- » No means NO. It is important to be able to trust the person you are playing with so make sure you respect their boundaries and remember that the 'no' in the negotiation stage means 'no' throughout playtime!

- » Drugs and alcohol. Lots of people like a drink or two to get into the mood, and some people like to engage in recreational drug use. I am not here to judge people's life choices, but consuming drugs and alcohol when playing really is not a good idea.

- » Informed consent. Always check and recheck — do you know enough about the play you are about to engage in? Has the person you are playing with consented to it? Are you both comfortable with the planned play? If the answer is no to any of the questions then don't do it!

» Keep it clean while you are being dirty! Keeping your toys clean is imperative. A simple antibacterial spray is useful on most toys, and if you are using insertable toys (vibrators, dildos, butt plugs, etc.) on more than one partner or on each other, cover them with a new condom each time you use them and always change condoms when inserting in an alternative orifice. Some people like to keep anal and vaginal toys totally separate and exclusive to avoid any mid-play mix ups and accidental cross contamination.

After all of that is done the next most important thing is to have fun.

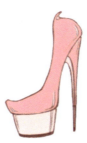

Taking Control

Taking control is all about one of you being Dominant and the other person letting go of the control. The words "Dominate me," "I want to be Dominated," or "I want to Dominate you" can sometimes obscure the core of "Domination." When stripped back to the most basic form, it simply means one person lets the other person take control. What they take control of depends on ground rules already discussed and agreed by both parties. If it still sounds all a bit confusing, then let's look at it another way; everyone "Dominates" or has been "Dominated" by someone at sometime. Have you ever been pressed or pressed someone gently into the bed whilst making love? That's a form of Domination.

Who takes charge? Well that's a negotiation between you and the person you are playing with - and that is the most important thing to remember — it's PLAY, and PLAY should be FUN! One of the most common problems I hear is when one partner is paralysed by "getting it wrong" and this fear takes all the fun out of playing. Once the mystery is stripped away you should be able to find your own style of Domination and have fun with it.

What is a Dom(me)?

Most people think of the whip-wielding, rubber clad bitch or the muscle-bound leather-clad drill sergeant when asked to describe a Dominant. In fact, a Dom (male) or Domme (female) can come in a million different forms. Further on in this guide, we will look at how you can find what sort of Dom(me) you are and how you can play that out in real time.

The Dom(me) — sometimes called a "Top" — is the person who is leading the play, the one in control. However, the carefully negotiated 'rules' actually mean that the Dom(me) is only the facilitator of the play, the guide so to speak. The submissive (sometimes called the bottom) is the one who gets to be played with in carefully negotiated boundaries.

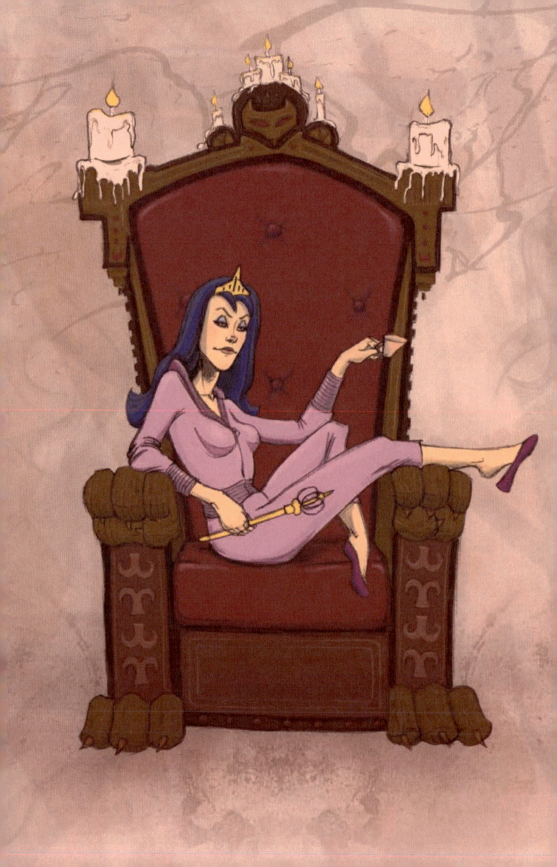

The D/s Relationship

It doesn't matter if you are a naturally more Dominant personality in day-to-day life or more Submissive. The roles you choose to play within your playtime do not have to reflect that part of your personality. Many people like to take on opposite roles of those they assume in day-to-day life, but that's not a fixed rule and neither is having to always play in one role or the other — don't be afraid to have a go at both the Dominant and Submissive roles.

First and foremost, the Sub/Dom(me) relationship is one of trust and respect. Without those attributes as a basic foundation, play becomes a dangerous game emotionally, and in some cases physically, so be careful to be open, honest and above all keep communicating with each other about how things are going.

The level to which this sort of play goes to is up to you and your partner but you may like to set up some boundaries around when play is and isn't appropriate; you may wish to let some of your games cross over into your day-to-day life but be careful not to bring day-to-day life into your play. For example, bringing anger about something your partner should have done, say the washing up, can break the play spell and leave you both frustrated and resentful.

The Care Involved

There is a lot of care involved in being a Dominant. It is important to remember the person in the submissive role is offering themselves as a gift to the Dominant. In short — don't break your plaything!

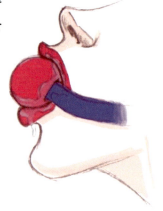

The Dominant may be getting what he or she wants, but the responsibility is a two-way street.

One very common mistake or misconception is that Domination is all about hate and anger when in fact in order to Dom(me) properly you have to take the utmost care and attention. Go through the rules and guidelines before you play and keep checking in with each other when you first start playing. It may seem a little lacking in fluidity at the beginning but once you find your groove it will seem like second nature.

Finally, before we look at what sort of Dominant you might be it is important to note that this sort of play very occasionally might bring up some deep seated emotional issues that you and your partner did not expect; such as memories of being bullied at school or parental confrontation. This is why it is important to have a safe word and communicate after the play to discuss anything that may have surfaced through the play.

If you decide to play in a Dominant role remember that it takes a lot of trust and courage to 'submit' so be mindful of that when playing. With the right approach, there is no need for sub/Dom play to be remotely intimidating — except as part of the fantasy play, of course. But before you reach for your handcuffs or whip, it's worth working out your preferred Domination style. It's not just what sex games you play that matters: it's the way that you play them too.

Style

It's very important to find your own style of Domination. People don't come in one shape or size, and neither do Dom(me)s. Part of the fun of creating a fantasy scene in your own bedroom is you can really be who you want during that time and the fun doesn't stop there because you can always change who you are next time you decide to play. Of course everybody needs a foundation, so let's start by exploring the things that *you* find Dominant.

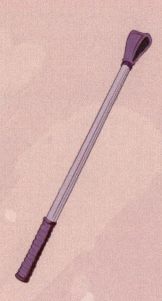

Chapter Two

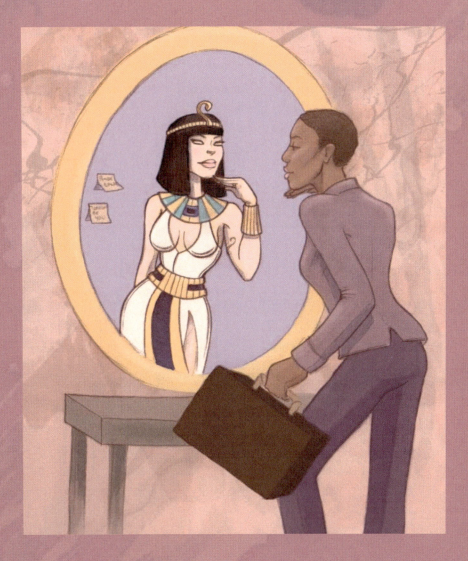

Finding your style of Domination

Dominant Character

Start out by thinking about people, historical figures or characters that you would consider as strong or Dominant and larger-than-life. Jot down the one or two names that pop into your head immediately.

These could be characters from your childhood, who captured your imagination like Wonder Woman or Batman. You may find that the first character that pops into your head is a historical figure whose story captivated you as a teenager, like Cleopatra or Robin Hood. Alternatively, you may find that someone from popular culture has inspired you recently like Lady Gaga or even Alan Sugar.

There is no right or wrong answer because everybody's inspiration and ideas of strength are different. Make sure you're not trying to think about what other people might consider strong or Dominant. You don't have to be anything like their age, size, nationality or even gender. This should be a personal choice — no matter how bizarre!

What is Dominant about them?

Now you have that person or character in your head start thinking about what it is you find so powerful and alluring about them. Take a moment to write down a list of those character traits.

Make sure that these are coming from you and not an idea of what you think others might find powerful and alluring. You might think that Beyonce is your top dominant person because of her independent nature, down to earth character and non-diva behaviour. Some of you may go for a James Bond-type character because he is suave, sophisticated and cool in dangerous situations. It's amazing the variety of different types of characters and people who come up when I ask this question.

One lady, when asked this question, chose Tinkerbell as her Dominant character because of the way that she dressed in pretty pastel colours, was small but strong and was the one that made Peter Pan believe in himself when nobody else did and never gave up. The Incredible Hulk was also a suggestion that somebody came up with as their Dominant, larger-than-life character because of the immense strength, perceived rage and yet gentleness to those who are doing good deeds.

Gender and sexual orientation should be no barrier when thinking of the character that you identify with. It's a fun thing to try out on your friends to see who they identify with!

Your Dominant Style

Now, using <u>their</u> character traits you can identify and develop your inner Dom(me). Now, I'm not suggesting that you paint yourself green if you identify with the Incredible Hulk, but think about what you find their most attractive features. They are probably the ones that you would like to emulate and will find the most easy to do so.

So if we take the Incredible Hulk as an example, you might like to use a quick change of total calm to (pretend) rage to unsettle your play partner to take control of the situation and therefore dominate the scene. If you chose Sharon Stone as your ultimate powerful alluring character the draw to her personality might be her use of overt sexuality and flirting, which she uses as a manipulative tool. Taking control and playing with domination is about putting aside everyday life and starring in your own movie!

Methods of Domination

Now that you have managed to find your inspiration it may be useful to see how individual your style is and how many other types of Dom(me) you could have chosen and can play with once you have explored your main Dominant character trait.

You can sum up your Dominant character's traits; take a look at some of the suggestions below which you could use to summarise their style:

The Princess Dom, the Prince Dom, the all action hero, the all action heroine, the cool calm assassin, the femme fatale, the rich bitch, the cocky tycoon, the evil Lord, the wicked Queen, the secret superhero, the boss, the free spirit, the tortured soul, the rock chick, the biker boy, the bully, the stripper, the spy, the tease, the manipulator, the strong silent type, the underdog, the gangster, the moll, the captain, the Emperor, the Lady of the Manor, the Lord of the Manor…

Which one did you identify with? You may be a mix of some of the above types. Of course this list is not exhaustive; these are just a few characters you could pull from in order to create your Dom(me) style or play with a different persona each time you play.

It's not about dressing up to look like one of these characters, it's about thinking what it is about that character that makes them so in charge, and then using that as a tool to create your personal, unique Dominant character. Feel free to give this persona a new name; even megastar Beyonce uses a character to bring out the "dominant" in her; she uses a character called "Sasha Fierce."

Now you have your stylistic starting point it's time to introduce the play... Walking into the bedroom head to toe in leather or latex whilst brandishing a whip is probably not the best way to gently introduce domination to your partner. Although it may seem boring, laying the foundations and ground rules before you start to play will mean more fun, more freedom, and less confusion... and did I mention more fun?

Chapter Three

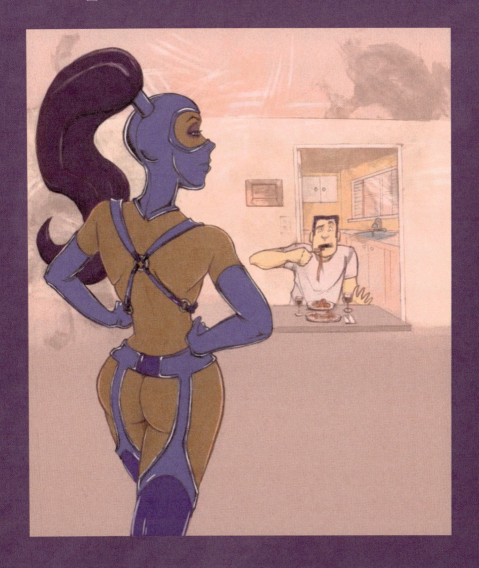

Introducing Domination into your relationship

If it is you that is introducing control and domination into the bedroom then just take a moment to clearly think about what you want to achieve without scaring the pants off the person that you are with (although the pants may be removed at a later date). You may have a very clear idea of exactly what you want to do in the bedroom in a controlling position, but jumping straight to that point may be five steps beyond what your partner can deal with at first. On the flipside if your partner is bringing up the subject remember that they may not have read this book and therefore may not have thought about a good way to ease the subject in!

Bringing up the subject

There are various ways of bringing up the subject yourself. However, I would advise against this kind of discussion in the throes of passion as it can knock your partner's confidence and trust. If you suddenly — in mid-intercourse — blurt out something like "I want to stick my foot in your mouth while you're lying on the floor trussed up like the Christmas turkey", odds are it's not going to have the desired effect.

A good way to introduce the subject is by proxy; kinky subjects are always being written about in magazines and newspapers. So find a topical story, and use it as a way to bring up the subject. For example "have you seen what filmstar X wore to the Oscars? It's very Fetish don't you think? I really like the style of it… Have you ever done or thought about doing anything like that in the bedroom?"—the discussion is now open! If your partner, flat-out says "No" then you can go onto stage two of asking if it's something fun they might consider having a go at.

If you're reading this book because your partner has brought up the subject of you taking control in the bedroom (or even bought you this book as a hint) there are some important things to remember. Firstly, just because one person is into it doesn't mean that you will be, or *have* to be, but remember; nothing ventured, nothing gained. And if they have brought up the subject it probably took a lot of courage for them to do so. Secondly, and most importantly, time between you and your partner should be FUN!

All too often I see terrified partners sitting in front of me at seminars or classes I teach because they have lost sight of the overall importance of the word "play." And lastly, although I would never advise you to do something you really don't want to, it may be that some of the stuff your partner suggests may not be 100% to your taste, but most people do find a delight in pleasing their partners, and so as long as you can make whatever you're doing fun, it's amazing how much you can get out of losing yourself in somebody else's game…

Who Plays Which Role?

There are no hard and fast rules about having to stay either 100% dominant or 100% submissive. In fact, a lot of people like to play between the two. Communication is key to any successful play. Once you have the initial conversation to introduce some form of domination and control in the bedroom, it's time to create some ground rules, which will be the foundation of every playtime. It's important to remember that sometimes things don't work, just like any kind of intimate play in the bedroom. The more you play, the more you get to know each other. And the more you get to know each other, the better the play will be.

It may be helpful to read the Absolute Beginner's Guide to Submission, if you think that you may like to switch roles, or perhaps read both guides together and use them as a talking point for negotiating the ground rules and deciding which role you want to play in first.

Re-read the 10 rules of conduct and go through each and every point and make sure that you are both clear on every aspect. It's just as important to cover no-go areas as it is to talk about things you would like to do, and even more important to respect each other's no-go areas.

Creating the ground rules

It may seem dull but creating ground rules is an important thing to do, even if you have known your play partner for years. It's very easy to stop communicating when you've been with somebody for a long period of time and it's actually quite a good exercise to rediscover each other. This can be an exciting and hot time together — just like when you first met!

Some people like to start off the play with some sort of ritual, and this may depend on how intimate you are already with your play partner. For example some people like to start by having their partner run a bath for them, bring them a glass of wine and layout a particular outfit in advance.

You may like to try a more symbolic start to your play by putting your partner in a leather collar, or if this is too "hard-core SM" for you the simple task of getting your partner to undress slowly in front of you works just as well. If this is a known start point for play then you both know that your rules of conduct apply from that point on. It's also a good idea to agree an end-point or signal too; this may be a time frame, word or something as simple as a kiss on the forehead.

Chapter Four

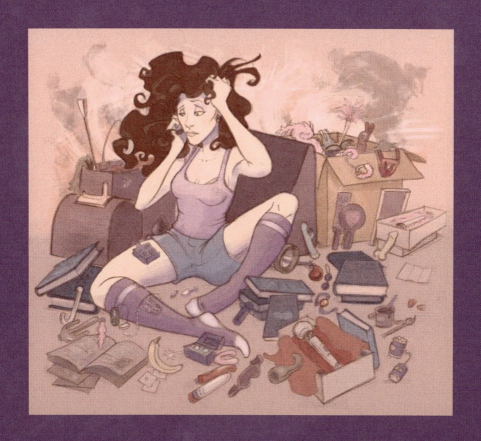

Equipment

Using Yourself!

You don't need to spend a fortune on the latest sex gadgets to play, because the most valuable piece of equipment you have is yourself! Think about how you use your voice, your body, and your touch. Anticipation can be just as effective as any cane or flogger. Try sitting your play partner down when naked, or semi-naked, and using your voice gently tell them what you would like to do to them in your play session.

Slowly walking around your play partner and getting very close with your body, but not touching them, is likely to make them very compliant. Silence is also very powerful and can put your play partner on edge and eager to hear what you want them to do next. Eye contact is also very powerful — fix their gaze for longer than seems natural to have them squirming in their seat

Basic toys

If you're ready to start putting a few items together for a play toybox, then think about what sort of play you and your play partner would like to engage in first; there's no point in spending hundreds of pounds on floggers if you and your partner are unlikely to use them in play. A simple blindfold can be a very effective tool when you start to play and this can be anything from an expensive silk version or just something to hand, like a man's tie.

Try repeating the anticipation game above, but with your partner blindfolded — taking away one sense will make all of the others heightened, but be sure that your partner is comfortable being blindfolded before doing so; being blindfolded takes a lot of trust and although the element of surprise is a good tactic, you don't want to make your partner so jumpy that they're not going to enjoy the play.

Other basic toys could include:

- Wrist cuffs — easy for restraint and many come in soft leather which is better for not leaving marks after play, unlike restraints like handcuffs!

- Dildos - Not everybody's cup of tea so check first that it is something that your partner is into or may like to try — and remember to use lots of lube.

- Vibrators — Good for boys and girls

- Rope — It's always good to read a basic manual on rope play before you get going.

- Pegs — A simple clothes peg placed on the nipples can heighten sensation, but remember, it hurts more when they come off than when they are on.

- Floggers — Whips with many strands attached to the handle. These can be used sensually as well as a 'punishment' toy!

- Paddles — These can really do some damage, so be careful and read up a bit on where it is safe to hit!

The key to collecting a basic box of equipment is to think carefully about what you and your partner really want to play with. Take it slow and ask questions about the equipment — which means you should be shopping in specialist stores or finding a local kink market, so you can talk to someone who really knows about the kit. Have an idea what is out there in the market before buying your next toy and have fun with your purchases, but also be prepared to make mistakes and upgrade toys as you go along.

It is also essential that you make sure you clean your toys carefully after you use them. Make sure you cover insertables with a condom, wash toys with a good antibacterial cleaner and spray toys that cannot be washed with a good antibacterial spray. It is also good to have a first aid kit to hand (just in case) and a pair of safety scissors if you are playing with rope.

Outfits and Fetish Fashion

You don't have to go the full hog and get dressed head-to-toe in leather or latex (unless you want to, of course), but sometimes a special item of clothing can help to put you and your play partner in the mood. Pick an outfit that makes you feel confident and sexy and fits the type of scene you're trying to create.

There are plenty of online clothing sites that sell everything from pretty lingerie to studded leather tops, so you don't even have to leave the house to play dress up. The main thing to remember is that an outfit is not going to be the key to you taking control, it can be an aid or a tool, but the Dom(me) has to come from within you, not from what you're wearing or what toy you're holding.

If you feel like you need an added boost to get into your Dominant character then try buying a wig that is very different from your own hairstyle. You will be amazed how different you can look and feel just by changing your hairstyle!

Chapter Five

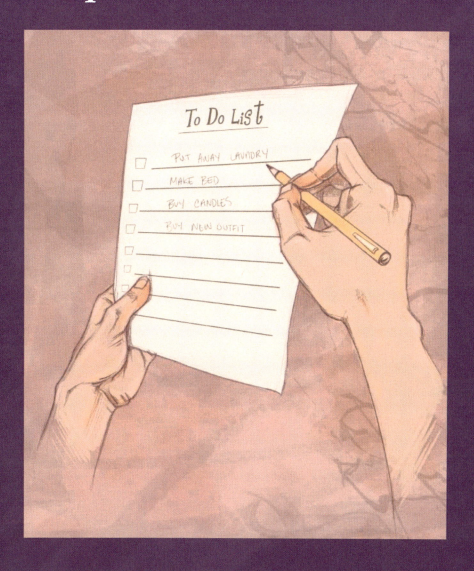

Games, Scenes & Planning

Now What?

So you have your Dom(me) style sorted, had the conversation with your play partner to find out what sort of play is acceptable to both of you, bought a few toys, found a suitable outfit that makes you feel sexy and confident, and set aside some time for play where you won't get disturbed by calls/kids/work. Now what?! Well, it's good to have a game plan for what you're actually going to do when you're playing with your partner.

Some people like to plan the entire play session from start to finish. This has its advantages and disadvantages, because it can make you feel secure in what you're going to do, but doesn't leave much leeway for spontaneity. To leave room for that spontaneity it's a good idea to have the start and the end of your play in mind and then have three or four sections that could be introduced in the middle. It's important to note that not all play has to end in sex — for some people this type of play is better than intercourse and this is something you should discuss with your play partner before you start.

An example

- » You have already decided that you're going to start the play in the bedroom with your partner waiting in there for you naked

- » You start by blindfolding them and leave them to anticipate what will happen next as you announce that they must sit still whilst you go and get changed in another room.

- » You know that your objective is to make your partner so hot for you that they will be trembling just to be able to touch you.

- » Your middle sections include the use of a pair of wrist cuffs, a double-ended clip (to clip the two cuffs together) and a soft flogger to run across their body.

- » You will use your voice and an occasional touch to describe what outfit you are wearing.

- » Your end game is for your partner and you to engage in sex.

So now you have an idea about what you want to start and end with, and what you want to have happened in the middle — it's time for you to put it all together.

Planning ahead

By planning ahead and having everything in its place ready for your play, it means that there is less stress on you trying to find things and you can just concentrate on your game plan. Using the same previous example (blindfold, entering the room in your new outfit, wrist cuffs, flogger, endgame = sex), it would be good to make sure that your outfit is complete and in another room for you to change as fumbling through drawers looking for something when play is supposed to have started is a sure-fire way to kill the mood.

Planning ahead also means thinking about how what you do will affect the other person; so before you get into your hot outfit in another room and before your partner is coming into the bedroom, it might be an idea to place the chair in the middle of the bedroom and have them sit on it and blindfold them, before you start.

Alternatively, if you want to be ready before they arrive you may leave the blindfold on a chair with a note saying "Undress, put this blindfold on, sit on this chair and wait." The blindfold means that while you are not in the room they can start thinking about what you might be wearing and what is going to happen without the distractions of looking at things in the room.

Using a blindfold also means you won't feel "stared at" while you start your play and you could even take in a few notes… who'd know with a blindfold on, eh?! When you are out of the room you need to think about the experience of the other person, so think about putting music on, but make sure it's the right type of music for the mood you are trying to create.

When you come back in the room think about the anticipation they already have by just hearing the door open. Plan ahead by preparing the first thing you're going to say to them. Remember, at this point your partner is likely to be quite nervous if they've been blindfold for while, and their first reaction may be to giggle. Think about how you're going to deal with this, and whatever you do don't take it personally. A lot of people's first reaction when they are nervous is to giggle.

If you put the cuffs on them while they are blindfolded their attention will be just focused on the feel of the cuffs. Clipping those cuffs behind your partners back means they are now in a position for you to whisper what you would like to do to them into their ear. You can also use your body to press into the back of their head and gently caress down the front of their body with your hands.

Take some time to describe your outfit; it may seem like millennia to you but that's because you're going to be thinking ahead — you need to let your play partner savour the moment and savour the vision in front of them. Now, you know your end game is to get them into a position where you can "use" them sexually, so leading them to the bed would be the next logical move.

You may then wish to take the blindfold off to let them see your outfit. In preparing for the moment when you reveal yourself think about how the room will look when they take the blindfold off; bright lighting is likely to dazzle and ruin the mood, so think about dimming the lights or putting some candles around the room. Also, if the room is cluttered with washing or children's toys that need putting away, it's not going to help you create your fantasy world for yourself or your play partner.

Think about whether or not you want to direct your play partner to get onto the bed by direction or whether you want to unclip their wrists and lead them gently to the bed yourself. And depending on how you're feeling right now you may wish your partner to kneel on the edge of the bed and pleasure you orally. Alternatively, you may wish to instruct your partner to lie on their back so you can attach your partner's arms above their head to the bed.

If you are thinking about restraining them as part of the play you may wish to attach pieces of rope to your bed in advance, so you don't have to think about how you can attach your partner's cuffs when you get there. If you don't have a bed where you could easily attach your partner's cuffs to, then one long piece of rope underneath the mattress works just as well — just attach the cuffs either side.

Now you have your partner in position think about taking some time to tease before devouring your partner. One of the biggest worries I hear about playing with partners and teasing is that people are afraid that their partners get bored. But think about it this way; if you enjoy a good massage you don't want it to be over the moment you are laid out on the massage couch, you want it to go on for ages! How long you tease for at this stage is up to you; seeing as you are the dominant it's your prerogative, but at this stage it is probably very obvious whether or not your partner is enjoying themselves!

Thinking up games, or using one of the eight suggested in this book, may need preparation. Sometimes it's great to let your play partner have an idea of what might happen in the session by asking them to do tasks prior to actually being in front of you. Suggestive hints or texts about what might happen are sure to pique your play partner's interest. And if you are preparing some time in advance you might like to start building this up days before your planned playtime.

Other things to think about when you are preparing are refreshments. You and your play partner might get thirsty and it's better to have a couple of glasses of water on standby so you don't have to rush to the kitchen mid-session! If you and your partner use condoms when having sex, or if you have more than one play partner and are using toys that are insertable, then have plenty of condoms at hand. Using rope?

Re-check your safety list; e.g. is a pair of safety scissors to hand. Is your partner asthmatic or on medication they need to take regularly? If so, have you made sure that it's in the room/nearby and you both know where it is!

Games to Get You Started

Once you relax into playing with your partner it will get easier to start thinking up scenarios and games. Here are eight ideas to get you started, but don't feel restricted to using these. Coming up with creative ideas is part of the fun!

Role-Play Challenge

Role-play is not for everybody, but some people like to be someone else when they play, as it makes it easier for them to step out of their everyday lives. Get your play partner to write down three different role-play duo characters (one dominant/one submissive). Put them in envelopes and number them 1 to 3; then get your partner to choose the number of the envelope the day before you play, and you can start putting together props or outfits that may come in handy for that particular role-play.

You could take this a step further by personally suggesting three role-play duos and get your partner to write a short fantasy about each one before picking the one that you would like to play with.

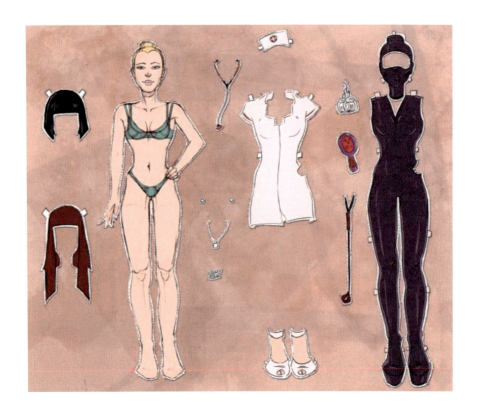

You don't have to tell them which one you've picked until they enter the room to play — unless you want them to prepare some form of attire for themselves that fits the role-play scenario. Role-play duo characters can be anything you like — for example, teacher and pupil, doctor and patient, Lord/Lady of the Manor and stable hand, etc.

Sex Quiz

It's amazing what sort of outrageous facts you can find on the Internet! Note down 10 questions and answers, and once you have your play partner in place (and possibly naked) you can ask your questions and decide the fate for those they get right or wrong. If you're going to allow your plaything to masturbate at the end of the play session perhaps the amount of questions they get right determines how many minutes they have to masturbate.

Alternatively, you could have 10 implements (a crop, cane, or just your hand) and any question they get wrong they get one stroke of the crop. If your partner is particularly into spanking then you could give them 1 minute spanking every question they get right.

Lotion in Motion

If you are happy for intimate interaction between you and your play partner then get them to really know your body by having them apply body lotion to every part of your body, gently massaging it in. Make it even more fun by having them blindfolded as this will make them more aware of every beautiful curve of your body.

Be aware that some lotions are not condom friendly so check the label on your chosen lotion before you start.

Roll the Dice

Purchase a cheap pair of oversized dice and then use sticky labels to change the numbers on one of the dice into tasks. For example; spanking, kissing, massage, etc. Then one of the dice becomes the action and the other dice becomes the length of time for that action or activity.

The fact that you're changing the dice to your own personalised tasks means you could actually ask your partner in advance the six things that they might like to have happen in session and then use those as a basis for your six sides of the dice.

Royalty for the Day

Play 'Princess Domme' for the day. If your play partner is particularly turned on by doing things to make you happy (which of course they should be) then you could suggest a royalty day where everything you ask (within prearranged agreements) is done for you and you get to be waited on hand and foot! Sometimes it's good to incentivise your servant for the day, and if you tell them what the reward is that they'll receive if they treat you like royalty that should make them work even harder!

Reward vs. Punishment

Negotiation is the name of the game here. Get your play partner to come up with five things that they would like to do in the play session. Get your play partner to do this well in advance, so you have time to think about things they have picked and they have time to think about how you might use that information.

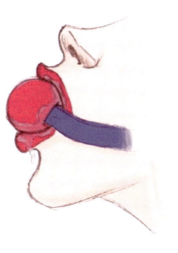

Being careful not to pick anything your play partner has set as a 'no go area' (see rules of conduct) match each of the things your play partner comes up with to a "punishment" that they would have to do to get what they want. For example, if your partner particularly likes you in stockings then you can set a task for them to do, like taking a minute of spanking, in order for you to put stockings on and for them to be able to see them.

If you know your play partner well enough, you can set the most challenging task for the thing you know they want the most.

Stranger Danger

To some people the thought of an illicit meeting in a bar is very exciting, but terrifying. Take out the actual danger by setting up a meeting in a bar with your regular play partner and pretend not to know each other. Then you can flirt and talk like it's your first date. Then, if your play partner behaves well enough, you may suggest that you take them home.

Prepare in advance by laying out certain play items that you know you and your partner enjoy playing with. When you get home and you have "captured" your date you can reveal what is waiting for them and then do with them what you will! If you are doing this type of role-play it's a good idea to make sure you have a very clear safe word in place.

It is also advisable to discuss how you might feel should your play partner be chatted up by other people while you are out and what you might do in that situation.

A little jealousy may be good to spark passion when you get back, but too much jealousy might result in waking the green-eyed monster and may have disastrous effects.

Clueless

This type of game takes some forward planning, but it can be very rewarding. After you have set aside a time to play, put together a set of clues for your partner. You could start with a clue about an item of play kit they need to pick up from a shop. Most specialist retailers will be happy to set something aside under a particular name. Get your play partner to go to the specified address and pick up the item you have set aside. Some retailers may be happy for you to leave a note in the bag which is to be picked up, or alternatively, instruct them to text you when they have picked up the item to get the next clue.

Don't make the clues too cryptic or your play partner may not understand what you want them to do. How long you make this erotically charged "treasure hunt," and where you take it, is entirely up to you. You could include a dinner rendezvous, hide clues around the house or give them a new clue every day for a week, which gives them the address to a hotel where you will be waiting for them to arrive along with your new toy.

Chapter Six

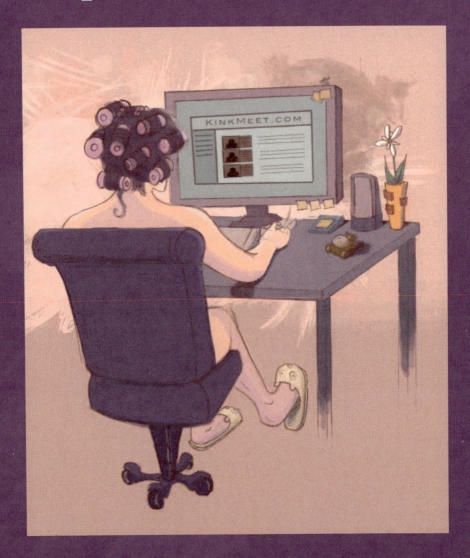

Out & About

Clubs and Events

Many cities and towns have social events; sometimes called munches. These are usually held in pubs and bars and are just casual social events where you get to meet people and can be a great way to develop a network of people who are open and friendly. You may be lucky enough to live in an area where classes are held for you to improve your skills. Some are better than others, and remember there is no formal qualification in teaching kink skills, so it may be advisable not to take everything said as gospel!

Lots of cities and towns around the world have regular kinky clubs, and Internet search should show if there are any in your area. Or look out for flyers in local kink and sex shops. Fetish and kink clubs come in all different shapes and sizes, so be careful to think about what type of club or event you might want to go to and do a bit of research online about the club.

Kink, Domination/submission and Fetish have become increasingly mainstream and much more widely accepted in general society, and when you start looking for like-minded people you will see that you are not alone!

Some clubs are more dressed-up and dance-orientated, others are more play-orientated, and some are more overtly sex-orientated. Do check the dress code before you go; a lot of fetish clubs require a minimum fetish or fantasy dress code. Most clubs have their own website and this will be clearly listed.

It may seem scary to go to a club the first time, especially if you're going on your own, but any well-run club should be welcoming and helpful. Lots of clubs have a "meet and greet" team who will be happy to introduce you to people. If you decide to take your play partner with you, you should remember that communication between you two prior to going out and during the night is key.

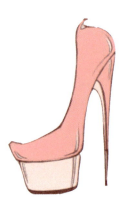

Finding a Playmate

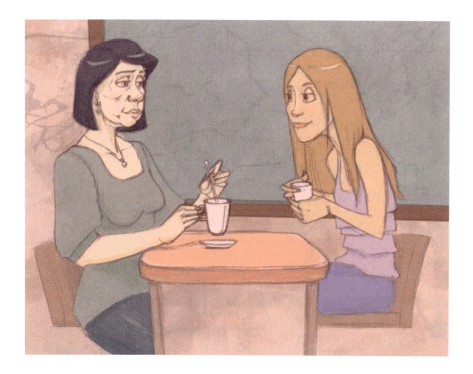

You may already be in a relationship where you can play, but not everybody is in that position. Just like any relationship, it may take time to develop your play side and it may take time to find a partner to develop that play side with.

A quick search on the Internet will bring up many different forums where you can find like-minded people, but as with any kind of Internet communication, you should be wary of meeting people outside of open public places and you should always err on the side of caution when meeting people for the first time.

If you are looking for a play partner and using the Internet or events to meet somebody, remember you don't have to play with the first person who communicates with you. Don't be afraid to ask questions of the person you're intending to play with, and don't feel any undue pressure to meet up or try something you don't want to try. The Internet is a great place to meet people, but keep in mind that it is also a place where sometimes people are not who they say they are.

There are lots of different types of relationships to be experienced on the scene, should you wish to do so. Many people find that once they start getting out and about, even if it is just out and about online, that there is a really amazing, supportive, fun kinky community out there in the world.

Further Reading

There are now hundreds of books on the market and lots of them available to just download on your iPad or Kindle. Have a look in your local kink store for books or check out online retailers like Amazon.com. While I would always suggest reading up on your chosen area of kink first, my best advice would be to get out there and have a go!

There are lots of local fetish websites and club sites, and many of them come and go. Some are more specialist, but here are a couple of the more established international sites of interest:

- www.FetLife.com — A bit like a fetish Facebook but you don't have to use your real name! There is lots of information on different types of fetishes and groups you can join online to find like-minded, local people should you wish to do so

- www.SkinTwo.com — One of the longest running kink magazines & now an online great resource for news, fashion and events.

- www.TheFetishistas.com - Online fetish magazine featuring latex, leather & rubber fashion, models, clubbing, news & events plus a directory

Annual Events

There are hundreds of weekly and monthly clubs & events around the globe. I have listed some links to the big annual events that are held worldwide, and have selected ones that are not orientated to any particular gender, sexuality or kink. There are, of course, many great events out there that cater to a more specialised audience for you to discover should you wish to…

European Annual Fetish Events

www.BoundCon.com (Germany)

www.German-Fetish-Ball.com (Germany)

www.LondonFetishWeekend.com (UK)

www.FetishWeekend.cz (Prague)

Annual Fetish Events (not location specific)

www.DommeTrips.com (Worldwide)

www.TortureGarden.com (various events around the world)

Australia & New Zealand Annual Fetish Events

www.OzKinkFest.com (Australia)

www.TheFetishBall.com (New Zealand)

USA Annual Fetish Events

www.DCFetishball.com (Washington DC)

www.DomCon.com (New Orleans)

www.DomConLA.com (Los Angeles)

www.FetishCon.com (Florida)

www.Fetish-Factory.com (Florida)

www.HalloweenBall.com (Nevada)

www.KinkFest.org (Oregon)

www.RubberBallUSA.com (Minnesota)

www.TesFest.org (New Jersey)

www.ThunderInTheMountains.com (Colorado)

Canadian Annual Fetish Events

www.FetishWeekend.com (Montréal)

www.VancouverFetishweekend.com (Vancouver)

Glossary

This is by no means a comprehensive list of terms you may come across in the fetish and kink world, but here are some of the more common words:

24/7: Acronym for 24 hours a day, 7 days a week. Used to refer to an SM or Dom(me)/sub relationship that is full-time.

Adult Baby Play: A scene where one participant takes on the role of a small infant and the other the role of the mother/nanny/aunt/daddy/babysitter/uncle. May or may not include genital sexual acts.

Age Play: Where one participant takes on the role of a child or teenager and the other the role of the mother/nanny/aunt/daddy/babysitter/uncle/teacher. May or may not include genital sexual acts.

BDSM: Acronym for Bondage and Discipline, Dominance and Submission, Sadism and Masochism.

Bottom: Used to describe the person in the more submissive role. Sometimes used if the 'bottom' would not consider themselves a submissive but likes being played with.

Breath Play: A term used to describe breath restriction in play.

D/s: Dominant and submissive play or lifestyle.

Dom: A male Dominant or Top.

Domme: A female Dominatrix or Top.

Edge Play: Used to describe dangerous practices that may have a life threatening "edge" to them or are associated with mortal danger.

Electrics: A form of stimulation using electric current. Can be used for pleasure or pain. Used below the waist.

Fem Domme: A female Dominatrix who believes in female supremacy.

Fetishist: Someone who is interested in fetish but may not be interested in the D/s powerplay.

Fireplay: Burning or play with fire. Usually done by the Dominant on the submissive.

Fisting: Where a hand (or two) is inserted in the anus or vagina.

Forniphilia: Human Furniture. The submissive is usually bound in very restrictive bondage and used as furniture (foot stool, table, lamp, etc.)

Hard Limit: The absolute no-go area for someone in play. This is respected by any responsible Dominant.

Hard Sports: Can sometimes mean scat play (faeces play) or can mean a range of the more extreme play, such as cutting & blood play.

Heteroflexible: A relatively new term. Used by those who identify as primarily heterosexual but will play/have sexual relations with members of the same sex from time to time.

Homoflexible: A recent term used by those who identify as primarily homosexual but will play/have sexual relations with members of the opposite sex from time to time.

Kinkster: A term used to describe someone who is into kinky things.

Medical Play: Includes medical procedures and implements. Usually includes one or more of the following; needle play, catheterisation, examinations, enemas, cutting, sewing.

Pansexual: Someone who is "gender blind" whose attraction to another person is not based on gender or sexual practice.

Perv: A term used by other "pervs" to describe each other. A "perv" is someone who engages in SM and or D/s play.

Play Piercing: Play where hypodermic needles or hooks are temporarily placed into the skin.

Playing: A term used to describe the time when two or more people engage in SM and/or D/s practices. It can also be used to describe specific practices e.g. pony play, knife play, etc.

Poly Relationships: A non-monogamous relationship.

Pony Play: The submissive assumes the role of a pony. Usually combined with the ritual of wearing elaborate "ponygirl" or "ponyboy" outfits.

Pro-Domme: A female who engages in SM and/or D/s practice for money and takes the dominant role. The male equivalent would be a Pro Dom.

Pro-sub: A person who engages in SM and/or D/s practice for money and takes the submissive role.

RACK: Acronym for Risk Aware Consensual Kink. Also see SSC.

Sapiosexuality: Someone attracted to, or sexually aroused by, intelligence and its use.

Scarification: Cutting or marking of the skin that is purposely designed to leave permanent marks.

Session/s: Time set for playing. A term usually used by Pro Dommes/subs.

SM: Sadomasochism.

SSC: Acronym for Safe Sane and Consensual. Also see RACK.

sub: submissive or bottom.

Swinging: Where primary partners engage in sexual acts with other people.

Switch: A person who plays both Domme and sub.

T-Girl: A male-to-female transsexual — may or may not include medical transformation.

Tie and Tease: A term used to describe a type of play which involves tying up and teasing a person. This type of play may or may not include total orgasm denial.

Top: Used to describe a Dominant. Sometimes used by those who do not wish to play in a D/s sense, but enjoy SM play.

TPE: Total Power Exchange. Where one person give up complete control.

Trampling: Standing on and "trampling" on another person.

Trans: A male-to-female or female-to-male transsexual — may or may not include medical transformation.

Vanilla: Used to describe those not in the scene. Boring, plain.

Watersports: Urophagia — play involving urine.

About the Author

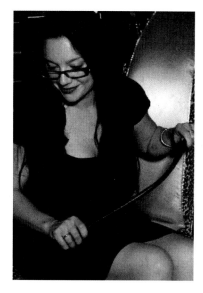

Mistress Absolute is a lifestyle and professional Dominatrix well known and revered worldwide. She holds a Masters in Gender, Sexuality and Culture and is often called upon to be a spokesperson for the kink community.

As well as training slaves, subs and servants for over 20 years she also ran one of the largest fetish clubs in the UK, 'Club Subversion' for 15 years.

An archive of her work to date is held at the Bishopsgate Institute, featuring her involvement with events such as the Skin Two Rubber Ball and FetishCon, as well as documenting her work as a Professional Domina.

Currently, she continues to run and co-ordinate one of the world's biggest fetish weekends, 'The London Fetish Weekend' and runs the bi-monthly event 'Club Femdom' as well as being involved in various other UK and international events.

She has appeared on BBC 1 and 2, Channel 4, Sky, Bravo and been featured in magazines including Loaded, Skin Two, Time Out & The LA Times. She models for various fetish sites, helps run a kink focused travel company 'Domme Trips', and occasionally performs at fetish events around the world.

Along with one-on-one sessions, Mistress Absolute also gives classes and tutorial sessions for couples and individuals wanting to know more about the fetish scene and kink.

Kink Education

www.AbsoluteBeginnersGuide.co.uk
www.MaxAbsolute.com

***

Clubs & Events

www.ClubFemdom.co.uk
www.LondonFetishWeekend.com
www.DommeTrips.com

***

Mistress Absolute's Websites

www.MistressAbsolute.com
www.AbsoluteBitch.com